Paleo for Restaurants

Don't lose customers when they reject grains and other neolithic foods

by Joe Disch

("Paleo Joe" of MadisonPaleo.com)

© 2014 Joe Disch

Also available as a Kindle® e-book.

To Beth, Bryn, and Emily -
who endure all my questions,
omissions and substitutions
when we go out to eat.

Contents

Disclaimer

I'm not a doctor or health professional of any kind, and I'm not telling you what to eat or what will make you healthy. At the time of this writing, I don't even operate a restaurant. I'm just one of millions who have enthusiastically adopted a "paleo" style of eating, and I'd like to help you understand how restaurants can better serve us.

The statements made in this book and related web sites have not been evaluated by the FDA (U.S. Food & Drug Administration). Products sold on madisonpaleo.com and servepaleo.com are not intended to diagnose, treat, cure, or prevent any disease. The information provided is not a substitute for consultation with your physician, and should not be construed as medical advice.

At the time of this writing, I am employed by Willy Street Co-op. Opinions expressed are my own, and are not necessarily shared by my employer. It should be assumed, though, that editorial bias toward Willy Street Co-op may influence some content.

Some links take you to external sites for more information. I do not necessarily endorse all such third party sites and am not responsible for their content. Some links represent affiliate relationships. If you purchase something as a result of visiting one of these links, I may receive a small commission.

About the author

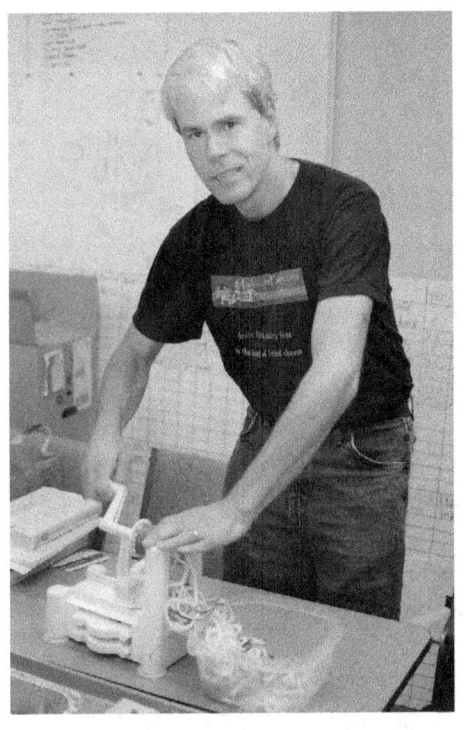

My name is Joe Disch. I live in Wisconsin, where seemingly every restaurant features fried cheese curds. I run the Madison Paleo web site, and I also work at the Willy Street Grocery Co-op, where I've presented multiple staff trainings on paleo/primal and grain-free eating. I'm not a nutritionist, restaurateur or medical professional.

I have studied the paleo diet extensively and have been happily following it since the end of 2011. I feel better eating this way than I did on the high-grain, high-soy, vegetarian diet I once believed in.

Think of me as an avatar for the growing ranks of frustrated paleo diners everywhere who want healthier options when we come to your restaurant. I'll help you understand what we're looking for, and how you can provide it without breaking the bank or alienating other customers. Basic paleo cuisine isn't rocket science. By definition it's so easy a caveman could do it. Let me be your guide in this return to ancestral eating.

What is paleo and why do I care?

According to a 12/17/2013 Huffington Post article, paleo was the most searched-for diet on Google in 2013.[1]

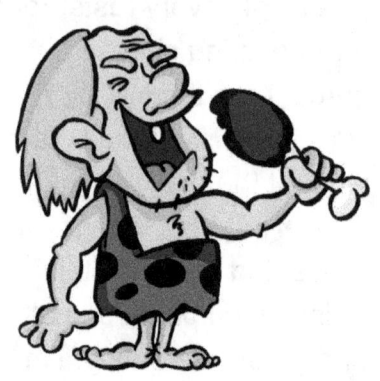

The paleo (or "paleolithic") diet is about eating whole unprocessed foods grown as naturally as possible. Plants and animals.

Though based on modern science, it essentially models how our hunter-gatherer ancestors ate. Pre-agricultural humans ate wild animals and seafood, organic (no other choice) vegetables, some fruit, eggs, nuts, etc. They did not eat large amounts of grains, dairy (ever try milking a wooly mammoth?) or legumes – all of which contain known gut irritants and digestive inhibitors. They didn't use refined sugars (unless you count occasional honey), salt, or artificial colors, flavors, preservatives, etc. Much has been written about this

---

[1]

http://www.huffingtonpost.com/2013/12/17/most-googled-diets-of-2013_n_4426726.html

by others, so I'll refer you to their books if you want to learn more about the "why" of paleo. The crux is that most of our evolution occurred before agriculture, and we're simply not well adapted to many of today's foods.

Paleo isn't "one size fits all." There are different flavors and interpretations, and the experts don't agree on all points. At its core, paleo means no grains/legumes/dairy/artificial or refined ingredients, and instead: lots of healthy fats, animal proteins and non-starchy vegetables. There is disagreement, however, about how much fruit, or how many nuts. Some versions allow some full-fat dairy products, especially when fermented as in yogurt. Some exclude starchy tubers. Some actually encourage up to 20% "cheating", and exceptions for coffee or occasional alcohol are widespread.

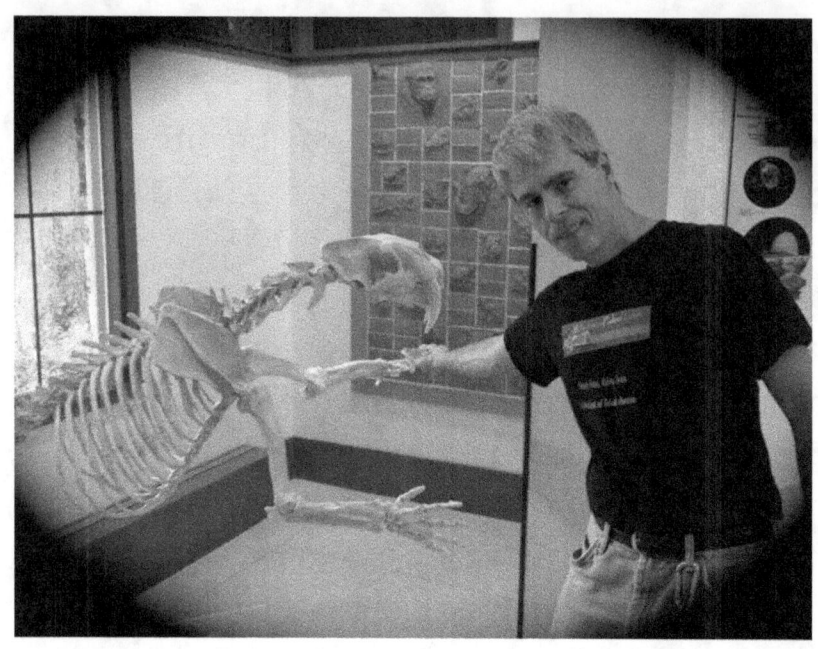

Almost no one wants to copy exactly what "cavemen" ate, even if it were possible. We've generally lost our taste for otherwise nutritious things like brains and insects, and many species of plants & animals have long since become extinct. The idea is to eat natural whole foods with the basic nutrition profile our bodies evolved (or were designed, if you prefer) to thrive on. Where you choose to go with this is ultimately your own decision.

What *we* see in your menu

Want a peek inside the mind of a paleo patron? Here are a few of our most common thoughts as we look over your menu for the first time:

"Steaks... that'll work."

We know we can probably construct an order based on real foods without being too annoying and/or defaulting to a salad. Maybe there's a simple vegetable side or other good options. If not, I can just have the meat and still feel like I've eaten. Here's hoping they don't use one of those "grill seasonings" with gluten in it.

"If nothing else, I can get a salad."

(See steaks, above) - This may be seen as an entree of last resort because it's been all too often the only choice. Even as such, you're going to have to endure my list of exclusions: "...hold the croutons, and the cheese, and can I just have a lemon wedge instead of dressing?"

"A burger would be good. I wonder if it's worth the hassle."

I'm still concerned about the grill seasonings, but more so about "extenders" like bread crumbs. Then, do I settle for a "gluten free" bun or risk a funny look for omitting the bun entirely? Will it be a problem to sub something for the fries? Maybe I'll stick with that salad.

"Oh I can't eat that - There's (gluten/dairy/sugar/whatever) in the sauce."

We skip right past most of your more creative offerings, knowing (or assuming) they rely on deal-breakers like wheat flour, milk, corn syrup, or whatever is personally non-negotiable.

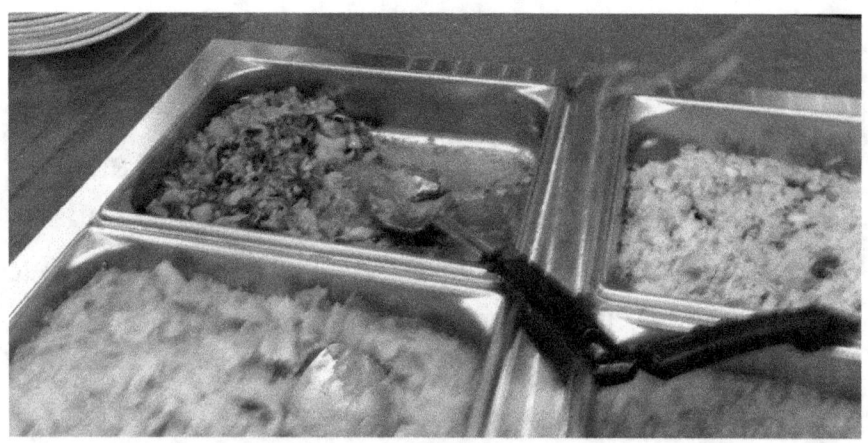

"That would be <u>awesome</u>... if it wasn't (probably) made with "x"

Sometimes our eyes stop on something really promising and we get excited - but then it hits us that it's probably "extended" with bread crumbs. Or fried in oil that's been cooking breaded things all night. Or the tempting cilantro lime sauce might be wheat-based. You get the idea.

What's the least I can do so Grok[*] can eat?

Are you perfectly happy with your current menu and clientele, but folks have mentioned they can't bring certain friends to your place because you don't serve anything they'll eat? You don't want to alter your vibe or add a bunch of new dishes, as your core customers seem to love things just as they are. A few painless tweaks could make you more paleo-friendly without requiring major changes:

→ **List your options on the menu and make sure staff understand them.** This includes "small" details like being able to order a sandwich "naked", or maybe lettuce-wrapped instead of on a bun.

→ **Have plain olive oil and/or lemon wedges available among your salad dressing options**, and/or a simple vinaigrette made with olive oil. Make cheese and croutons "opt-in" rather than "opt-out".

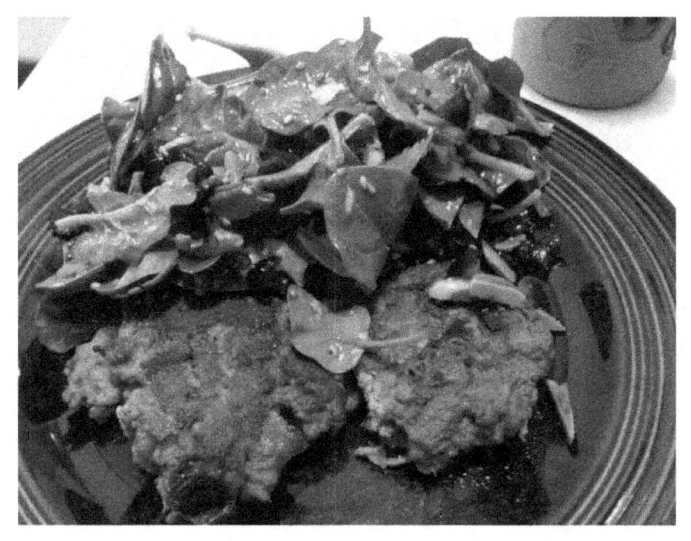

→» **Consider offering one paleo option (ideally not a salad) and include "paleo", "primal", or "caveman" in the title** so it will jump out at those who care. ("Paleo Plate", "Primal Dinner", "Caveman Special", etc.) It should be a <u>simple meat dish</u> with an <u>extra-large portion of non-starchy vegetable/s</u> (organic if you can.) **No potato, bread, pasta, beans or peanuts.** Sauces (if any) should be clearly identified as <u>free of any dairy (butter, cream, milk, cheese, etc.), refined sugar, grains (flour, cornstarch, etc.) or anything artificial like MSG. Use (and mention) only olive, coconut, or animal oils in this dish.</u> **We understand it may cost a little more.** Bonus points for wild/grass-fed meat and/or organic vegetables.

→ **Paleo also works for <u>some</u> people avoiding gluten** due to Celiac disease or other sensitivities, following low-carb diets (Atkins, etc.), managing peanut and soy allergies or lactose intolerance, and various other special needs. However, it is important to note that certain individuals' needs will not be met by any less than meticulous adherence to protocols you may be unprepared to ensure. Be sure you don't make promises you can't guarantee. ("*Gluten free*" for example, is a very strong statement involving legal standards often misunderstood.) On the other hand, one or two thoughtful paleo options, properly labeled and fully understood by staff, will really make your restaurant stand out to a large, fast-growing, and largely frustrated population.

---

* "Grok" is a fictional character representing the modern hunter-gatherer, created by Mark Sisson of *Mark's Daily Apple* (see blog list.)

The next step - level up with better options

Want to go a little further? Beyond simply "workable" to someplace paleo diners actually look forward to? For that you'll need to kick it up a notch, offering at least one home run paleo dish, and tightening things up a bit so as many of your remaining dishes are acceptable as possible.

The first part is actually pretty simple. There are so many good paleo cookbooks and recipe sites out there, inspiration shouldn't be a problem. The slightly trickier part is limiting use of unwanted ingredients as much as possible. Avoiding gluten is the obvious starting point, but to really impress you'll need to reconsider the oils and fats you use, preparations with grain/dairy/legume ingredients, use of refined sweeteners, and perhaps the sourcing of your meats. It's really not that hard, though. **Whenever you're making (x) why not remove/change (y) so it's also paleo (Gluten free, low carb...)?**

Six simple substitutions

1.   **Oils** - Top choices for cooking are **lard** or **tallow** (especially if grass-fed) or **coconut**. **Olive oil** is also a good choice for raw use, such as in salads. If you're shooting for primal (which allows full-fat dairy) rather than paleo, butter is a good option, again better if grass-fed and even more so if clarified (ghee). **Avoid all seed/industrial oils (particularly when hydrogenated) such as soy, canola, corn, cottonseed, margarine, vegetable shortening**. Yup, the cheapest and most widely available are the worst - even the ones that have been promoted as "healthy." (Does this really surprise you?)

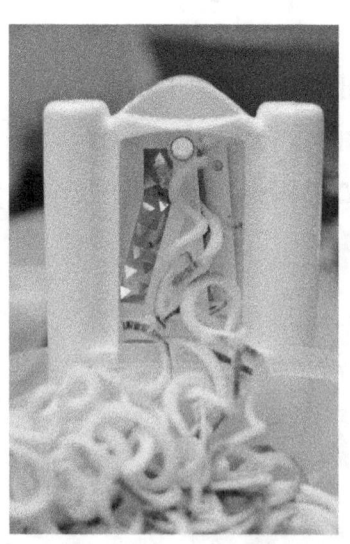

2.   **Zoodles** - Traditional pasta is out, but won't be missed if you get a spiralizer and make gluten-free, low-carb "noodles" out of zucchini, carrots or other veggies. These are cheap, super easy, remarkably

versatile, and surprisingly delicious. Process ahead, salt and drain. Then do a quick sauté as orders come in. Garlic & oil would be a good choice, or top with any appropriate sauce.

3. **Soy sauce** - Soy is generally avoided. Some people will accept small amounts of *fermented* soy (like soy sauce) **if it is wheat free**, but best to avoid it entirely or offer on the side. Try coconut aminos instead, or just season with sea salt. If must use soy sauce, at least choose a wheat-free tamari style.

4. **Sweet potato fries** (or turnip, parsnip, carrot...) - Some of us will eat "regular" (white potato) french fries, especially if cooked in a healthy fat like lard or coconut. **Sweet potato fries**, however, are more universal and are the preferred way to go! Either way, make sure any coating is free of wheat or gluten of any kind, and use a fryer that is never used for anything containing these. (Or coat with oil and bake.) If at all possible, make them yourself, using only the tuber/vegetable. That way you know there's no coating.

5. **Sauces** - If you currently serve any sauces based on wheat flour, try using something

else. Just subbing something like coconut flour could instantly put multiple dishes back on the menu for paleos and celiacs alike, and you just might be pleasantly surprised by the finished product. Even corn starch would be a big improvement for many people, and there are better options for compromise: arrowroot, potato starch, etc. Each has different properties, however, and it will probably take some experimentation to get it just right. Similarly, you could easily replace dairy in many sauces with coconut milk. Not always, but enough to justify a little tinkering. And for heavens sake, **stop hiding sugar in everything.**

6. **Vegetables** - You *think* you have vegetables on your menu, but we may not see them as such. First, I'm sorry to tell you that corn is a grain, not a vegetable. (Medleys, I'm looking at you.) Potatoes don't count either. Second, please refrain from covering your only vegetable option in cheese. Or cream sauce. Finally, vegetables are pretty cheap and filling. Give me a big pile of them, not a glorified garnish! Five a day was meant as a starting point, not an upper limit.

Going all the way
100% paleo restaurant?

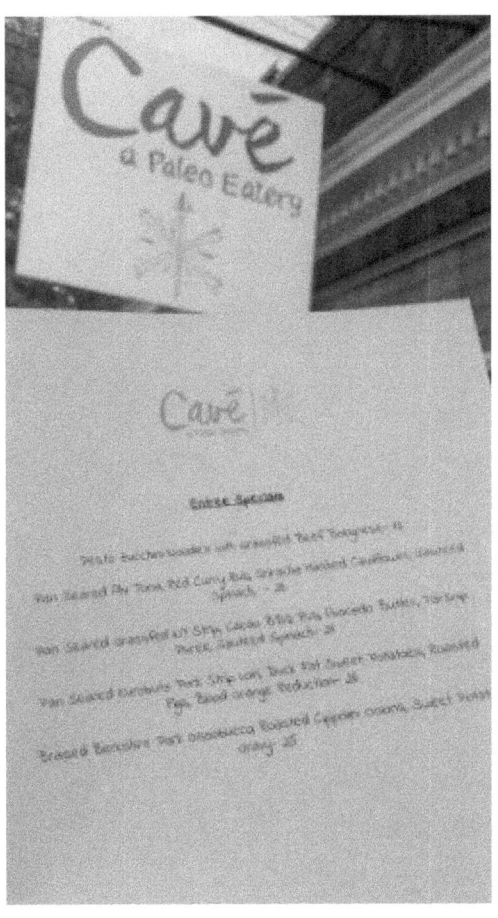

At the time of this writing, there aren't many entirely paleo restaurants. I know of a couple in Europe, a few in western states and another in New Jersey, and a couple food carts. I've no doubt this landscape will soon be very different. If you want to jump ahead of the curve, you'll need to go beyond "first aid" and perform some major surgery on your menu. This isn't necessary for everyone, but if you want to be a **destination** for the paleo crowd in the face of growing competition, you'll need to offer a variety of creative dishes (if not a whole menu) following <u>all</u> the rules.

We're talking grass-fed meats, healthy fats, organic ingredients when feasible, and no cross-contamination - at least with regard to gluten. A startup in Berkley (Mission Heirloom) is currently working on a franchisable cafe concept that does exactly this and more.

Some early adopters

Dine-in restaurants

Cavé - A Paleo Eatery, Avon-by-the-Sea, NJ
https://www.facebook.com/CavePaleoEatery

Sauvage, Berlin, Germany
http://sauvageberlin.com/en/

Palaeo, Copenhagen, Denmark

http://strictlypaleoish.com/palaeo-primal-lunch-in-co
penhagen/

Blooming Beets, Denver, CO
http://www.bloomingbeets.com/

Dick's Kitchen, Portland, OR
http://www.dkportland.com/

Paleo Cafe, Cairns, Australia
http://paleo-cafe.com.au/

Food trucks

Cultured Caveman, Portland, OR
http://culturedcavemanpdx.com/

Urban Caveman, Milwaukee, WI
http://urbancavemantruck.com/

Not So Fast, San Diego, CA
http://notsofastfoodtruck.com/menu/

Caveman Truck, Indianapolis, IN
http://www.cavemantruck.com/food

Outside the Box, Seattle, WA
http://www.eat-otb.com/

Caveman Cafeteria, Denver, CO
http://www.cavemancafeteria.com/

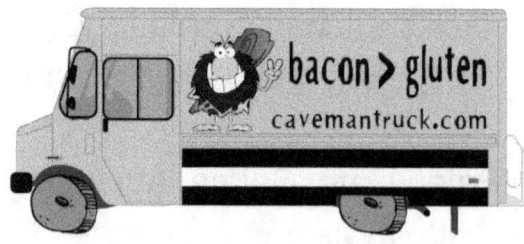

A few main course ideas
(beyond salads & naked burgers)

- **Sweet potato hash** - with sausage, ground beef, duck, leftover whatever
- **Steak (or other featured meat) and a baked sweet potato**
- **Beef stew (lamb, pork, elk, whatever...)**
- **Shrimp & zoodles** (zucchini pasta - quick sautéed on order)
- **Plantain wrap tacos**
- **Herb-crusted salmon and roasted asparagus**
- **Pork chops** - what ever happened to these?
- **Liver & onions** - just skip the flour dredge
- **Grass-fed burger between portobello mushroom caps** instead of bun
- **Thai chicken coconut curry**
- **Bacon-wrapped meatloaf and mashed parsnips**
- **Almond flour pancakes with sausage**
- **Paleo pizza on plantain crust**

It really doesn't have to be complicated. You can get tremendous mileage from creative pairing of a meat and one or more vegetables, seasoned in different ways. Pick a meat, pick a vegetable, pick your seasonings, done. Better yet, let the customer pick these from a list.

What about my profit margin?
(beverages and desserts)

You're not alone if much of your income flows from alcoholic beverages - and/or desserts, neither of which figure prominently in most people's idea of healthy paleo eating. However, many people embrace some form of paleo diet and still make room for occasional well-chosen indulgences. This could be an exception for wine with dinner, or a "paleo-ish" dessert on special occasions, or even a weekly "all bets are off" cheat day. For the rest (or if you're taking a more purist approach) flesh out your drink list with enticing preparations of seltzer, mineral water, teas (perhaps coffee), coconut milk, etc.

Paleo treats

Paleo treats and desserts often use honey, stevia, or maple syrup instead of more processed sweeteners, and/or may rely more on fat than sugar for their richness. They are nevertheless intended for occasional consumption only.

So many of these have been created as to become a running joke to many and an annoyance to others. You'll find tons of inspiration in paleo cookbooks and recipe sites. Some examples of what you might find:

- flourless paleo chocolate cake
- almond-flour paleo donuts
- coconut milk ice cream
- paleo chocolate chip cookies
- sweet potato brownie bites

If there's a paleo bakery nearby, you can probably outsource production of any dessert items you wish to carry, though some recipes for house-made treats are surprisingly simple to make.

Other dessert alternatives

- fruit (whole, baked, fruit salad, etc.)
- dark chocolate (perhaps house-made 90% cacao truffles)

Nonalcoholic drinks

- **nonalcoholic ferments**: kombucha, beet kvass, etc.
- **club soda** (soda water, seltzer)
- **mineral water** (still or sparkling)
- **teas**: green, herbal, other (maybe black, kind of a gray area)
- **bone broth** (ideally house-made)
- **vegetable juices**: carrot, cucumber, beet, spinach, kale...
- **fruit juices**
- **smoothies** (coconut milk is a great add-in, or even coconut oil if properly blended)

General beverage tips:

Offer optional add-ins: lime wedges, ginger twists, splashes of fruit juice, etc. Just make sure they're real and not the sugar & chemical laden kind sold for bar use.

If offering dairy (milk, cream, kefir...) choose some combination of full-fat, grass-fed, organic, raw and/or fermented. Avoid those with additives like carrageenan.

Alcoholic drinks

Alcohol is another gray area. Few would say it's "really" paleo, but many chose to drink it anyway. (One could construct plausible scenarios of various natural ferments, if one felt the need…)

Key points to remember are: definitely no gluten (most beers), ideally no grains (though little is left of what makes grains problematic), no added sugar or artificial ingredients. There are whole books of "paleo" cocktails, but my simple recommendations include:

Wine, especially red (again, organic ideal)

The Norcal margarita, or other tequila drinks (ideally 100% agave)

Mead (an ancient fermented honey beverage)

Coffee and coffee drinks

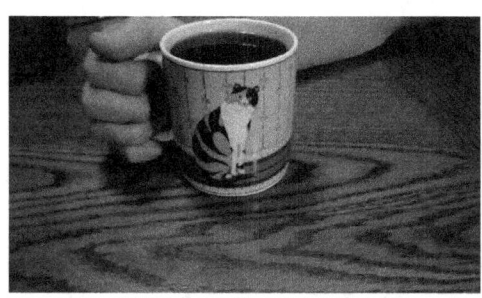 Coffee is a "gray area" food, embraced by some but shunned by others who say it's not paleo. For many, it comes down to quality. Organic will do better than conventional, and I'd say that goes double for add-ins like cream. If you're offering dairy, be sure **full-fat heavy cream** is a listed option. (Bonus points for organic and/or grass-fed.)

Many coffee shops now provide alternative milks for those who avoid all dairy, often soy (unfortunately), or almond, and occasionally (hooray!) coconut milk. This is far from universal, however, and I'm not alone in sometimes travelling with my own coconut milk. If you serve coffee, coffee drinks, or tea you'll make some big fans by offering this alternative.

It's not hard to find coconut milk in convenient refrigerated cartons or aseptic packages, any of which might suffice. If you want to be a paleo superstar, the extra mile would be using a canned full-fat coconut milk without additives. Just remember to mix before each use as it will separate. Shelf life is also shorter, usually about 3 days.

This is definitely extra-credit territory, but the ultimate gourmet option would be house-made- still easier than it sounds. Just blend coconut with pure water in a high-speed blender (such as a Vitamix®) and strain through cheesecloth.

"Enhanced" coffee

An interesting twist on full-fat that's become incredibly popular in some circles is buttered, or "fat-enhanced" coffee. Grass-fed butter and/or other fats are blended into hot coffee, creating a frothy mixture relished by bio-hackers, intermittent fasters, and those eating ketogenic.

"Bulletproof® coffee" (www.bulletproofexec.com) is the trademarked name (*Better Baby, LLC*) of a specific recipe including:

- At least 2tbs Kerrygold grass-fed butter
- 1-2tbs of MCT oil (not coconut oil)
- 2 cups of hot coffee brewed with low-toxin beans (like Bulletproof® Upgraded Coffee)

The term is sometimes misused in reference to any fat-enhanced coffee. Variants are being made with different combinations of ingredients. In many locations, Starbucks will blend Kerrygold butter into your coffee on request. This might be something you'd want to consider doing as well. An immersion blender works great for this.

Gluten, the #1 deal breaker

Understand that **true paleo also works for some people avoiding gluten** due to Celiac disease or other sensitivities, following low-carb diets (Atkins, etc.), managing peanut and soy allergies or lactose intolerance, and various other special needs. However, it is important to note that certain individuals' needs will not be met by less than meticulous adherence to protocols you may be unprepared to ensure. Be certain you don't make any promises you can't guarantee. ("*Gluten free*" for example, is a very strong statement involving legal standards often misunderstood.) On the other hand, one or two thoughtful paleo options, properly labeled and fully understood by staff, will really make your restaurant stand out to a large, fast-growing, and largely frustrated population.

Gluten is, to put it simply, a protein found in wheat and certain other grains which causes a range of health problems in certain people. These can be minor in some and very severe in others. (Some experts say it's no good for any of us.) Damage can be done by even a small amount of flour spilled on a dish, potentially starting a chain reaction that can last for months. Therefore, there is a big difference between not cooking with it and ensuring there is none in the food. If there's flour and dough flying everywhere in your busy pizzeria, I think the best you can offer is a "made without gluten" crust option, not "gluten free." (See the difference?) This is worth doing, but realize it won't be good enough for everyone.

Another tip from recent personal experiences: If someone asks to omit croutons from a salad, for example, don't throw on a side of bread instead! (At least not without asking first.) Because of the low margin of error with gluten contamination (seriously, a crumb is enough in some cases) any requests or questions regarding wheat or wheat products must be taken very seriously.

What about dairy?

Pardon the pun, but the paleo diet is... evolving. As good scientists, many early proponents of the lifestyle have tweaked their recommendations as new information became available. For example, exclusive use of lean meats has given way to embracing more fat, at least when sourced from healthy pastured animals. Directives to cut salt have softened. Canola oil, once promoted by some as a good choice is now understood by most to be another undesirable seed oil. You'll see widespread controversy about butter, white potatoes, and other foods. Additionally, there are different "flavors" of paleo; divergent philosophies and differing individual goals. There may never be agreement on whether paleo is necessarily low carb, or is what Robb Wolf calls "macronutrient agnostic." Arguably, one of the biggest divides is on the subject of dairy.

Paleo is generally understood to exclude dairy products, along with grains, legumes, seed oils, and anything artificial. It certainly seems unlikely that hunter-gatherers tried to restrain and milk mastodons. Perhaps more to the point, dairy products have been associated with a plethora of neolithic health concerns involving digestion, gut health, inflammation, and skin problems. Most of the world's adult population is unable to properly digest milk sugar (lactose) and/or protein (casein). Still, high quality dairy can provide valuable nutrients, and fermentation can blunt some of the digestive issues.

An ancestral type diet that includes dairy is often referred to as "primal" and is a popular variant. For our purposes this includes anything from full acceptance of dairy products down to only pastured ghee now and then. A typical profile might be: eschewing all mass produced dairy products but eating freely of pastured (perhaps raw) milk, cream, butter, and yogurt/kefir. The key point for a restaurateur is that there are many variations, and you'll need to decide how restrictive you want to be. Are you going for "pure paleo" (no dairy), mostly paleo with primal options, mostly primal with paleo options, or are you sticking with "traditional food" (named with the same irony as "conventional" produce) and just looking to offer paleo/primal options to patrons who are interested? This decision will determine some of your baseline practices, such as choice of cooking oils, and whether you need separate cooking utensils for different meals. I like to say that paleo is the new vegan, so it's kind of like choosing to open a vegan restaurant, a vegetarian restaurant, or a "regular" restaurant with vegetarian options on the menu. All can be successful, but your identity will shape your clientele, strategy, practices, and expectations.

Thanks to the lobbying efforts of the dairy industry, we've been taught from an early age that milk is a necessary part of our diet, primarily so we get enough calcium to grow strong bones and teeth. Trouble is: it's not the only, or even the best, source of calcium (and other essential minerals), and lactose can promote tooth decay much like other sugars. A diet rich in leafy green vegetables and bone broth might serve better in these areas. Dairy can, however, offer harder to find (and critical for health) vitamin k2, and a variety of healthy fats. This really only applies, however, if the milk is from grass-fed (pastured) cows, and is as minimally processed as possible. Raw milk is thought to contain the most nutrients of all, but is often hard to find because government regulators in many areas have outlawed it as potentially unsafe.

Cultured dairy foods such as yogurt and kefir reduce or eliminate problematic lactose and can be a good source of probiotics ("good bacteria") for gut health. Here again, quality is key. Typical grocery store yogurt is made from "factory farm" milk, with few strains of microbes and loads of sugar. Fortunately, alternatives are getting easier to find, and it's actually quite easy to make your own if you'd like to try that route.

If you'd like to include butterfat while minimizing lactose and casein, clarified butter or ghee may be your answer. This is made by melting and straining butter to remove solids. When made from pastured butter, this gives you all the good without most of the bad. Many otherwise strict paleo folks will make an exception for grass-fed ghee. (Many, not all.) The next step down on the "compromise ladder" would be heavy cream. This does include some solids, but far less than liquid milk and most other milk products.

If you're going to offer dairy products to this crowd, you might as well bake in the additional cost of organic. You *may* have trouble sourcing grass-fed (though it's important to try) but "conventional" milk will definitely be a deal breaker for many. Organic will avoid most of the added hormones, pesticides, and other chemicals used not only in the dairy but in the growing of the cow's feed.

Fats and oils

You might be surprised how important "good" fats are in the paleo diet. **"Bad" fats, on the other hand, are one of the main reasons we avoid eating out.** You're probably used to cooking with some kind of "vegetable oil", either liquid soybean/corn/canola oil, or a partially hydrogenated product made of these. I put "vegetable oil" in quotes because they don't really come from *vegetables*. Those in the know refer to these as industrial seed oils (also including sesame, sunflower, cottonseed, and others) and we see them as a toxic brew of extremely unbalanced fatty acids, chemically altered, unstable, and dangerously oxidized. Check any good paleo book for a detailed explanation of the myriad problems with these undesirable fats.

If you want to be taken seriously as a paleo chef, **switch to more natural choices like lard, tallow, or coconut oil.** If you're going for primal, butter or ghee are additional options. (Some paleos will also do ghee, since there's essentially nothing left but pure butterfat.) Further good options include palm oil and nut oils (but not peanut) though these are expensive and may add incompatible flavors. A good olive oil is fine for liquid applications that don't involve high heat. Don't forget about other ways to include healthy fats, like avocados, macadamia and other nuts, and yes bacon!

If you use peanut butter, consider offering almond (or some other real nut) butter instead. It's healthier and, not being a legume, is paleo friendly. Many people also think it tastes better.

Recipes

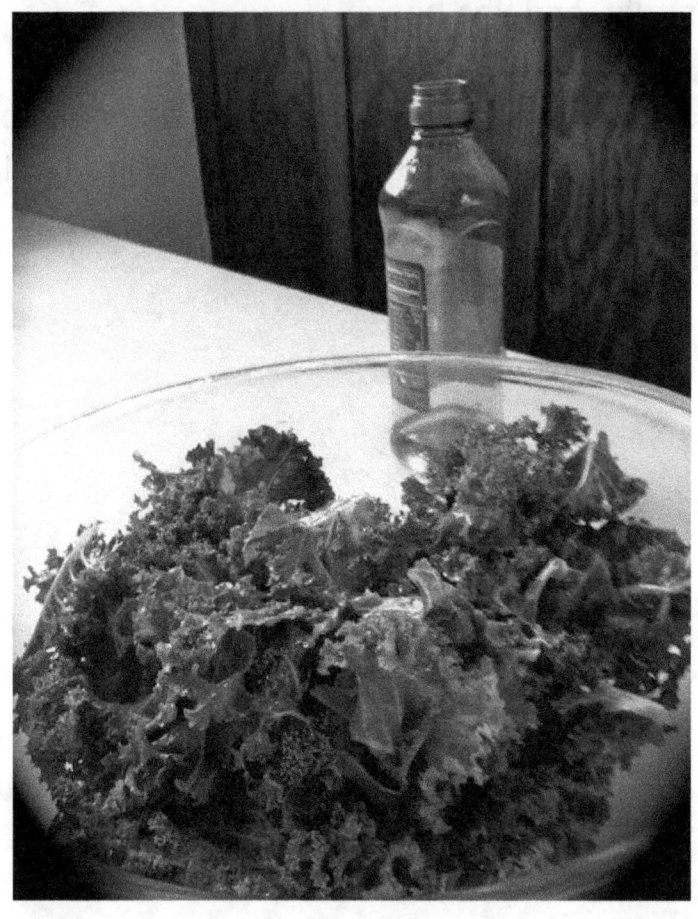

Paleo Joe's Kale Chips

1. Preheat oven to 350° F.

2. Roughly tear kale (preferably curly) into chunks or strips as it naturally comes away from the stem. Somewhat uniform is best but no need to obsess.

3. Wash in cold water, and <u>dry completely</u> using a salad spinner or paper towels.

4. Coat evenly with olive or melted coconut oil by drizzling then massaging with fingers.

5. Arrange in a single layer on baking sheet/s, preferably lined with parchment.

6. Turn off oven as soon as the chips go in. Use existing heat to bake for 10-20 minutes. (Time will vary considerably depending on your kale, your oven, and size of chips.) They're done when crispy but not burned.

7. If desired, sprinkle with any combination of salt, cumin, curry, garlic powder, cayenne, or whatever you like.

Plantain Wraps

Can be frozen but best warm & fresh from the oven

3 Green plantains • 1 cup water
1/3 cup extra virgin olive oil • 1 tsp. sea salt

1. Heat your oven to 375 degrees. Peel and chop your green plantains. It should come to 4 cups of cubed plantains.

2. Place all the ingredients in your high speed blender. (See below for food processor instructions.)

3. Using the tamper to push the ingredients into the blades, puree until it is smooth.

4. Spread on a parchment lined baking sheet. My baking sheet is 17" by 13" approximately.

5. Bake for 25-30 minutes, until it puffs a little.

6. Cut it into 6 pieces:

7. Stuff with whatever fillings you wish!

Reprinted with permission from Mary Lapp
at *Simple and Merry*

http://simpleandmerry.com/blog/aip-plantain-wraps/
https://www.facebook.com/SimpleAndMerry

Resource guide

Selected introductory BOOKS about paleo diet

Practical Paleo by Diane Sanfilippo

The Paleo Solution: The Original Human Diet by Robb Wolf

Everyday Paleo by Sarah Fragoso

Selected RECIPE SITES

www.paleoplan.com

http://paleomagonline.com/paleo-diet-recipes/

www.civilizedcavemancooking.com

www.pinterest.com/greenhsv/paleo-snacks/

www.paleomg.com/

www.paleofood.com/appetizers.htm

www.nomnompaleo.com/recipeindex

Selected WEB SITES about paleo diet

everydaypaleo.com

marksdailyapple.com *

robbwolf.com

ultimatepaleoguide.com

paleoleap.com

thepaleodiet.com

nomnompaleo.com

madisonpaleo.com **

paleodiet.com

chriskresser.com

civilizedcavemancooking.com

latestinpaleo.com

* primal
** author of this book

Selected Paleo COOKBOOKS

Everyday Paleo Family Cookbook

The Paleo Approach Cookbook

Everyday Paleo Around the World: Italian Cuisine

Everyday Paleo: Thai Cuisine

Paleo Magazine Readers' Favorites Cookbook

The Zenbelly Cookbook: An Epicurean's Guide to
Paleo Cuisine

The Primal Blueprint Cookbook

Paleo Indulgences: Healthy Gluten-Free Recipes
to Satisfy Your Primal Cravings

Gather, the Art of Paleo Entertaining

Paleo Comfort Foods

Paleo Happy Hour: Appetizers, Small Plates &
Drinks

Tools of the trade - equipping your cave kitchen

Essentials in most paleo-friendly kitchens:

- **spiralizer** - for making "zoodles" and other all-vegetable noodles
- **stainless steel, glass, and/or cast iron cookware** - these are inert and won't leach undesirable metals or chemicals into food like other options
- **slow cooker and/or pressure cooker** - for making certain meats, stews, and bone broth
- **glass food storage containers** - most plastics can leach various chemicals into food

One place to find them: www.servepaleo.com

A few new pantry staples:

- **coconut oil and/or pastured lard** - your new cooking oils
- **coconut milk** - for curries, soups, coffee, smoothies
- **coconut aminos** - wheat-free, soy-free alternative to soy sauce
- **pastured eggs** - a local farmer might value a plug on your menu
- **almond and/or coconut flours** - for paleo baking
- **real sea salt** - naturally sourced, includes a variety of minerals

Ask your vendor, find a food co-op, or try
www.servepaleo.com

Special offer:

Get a window sticker like this:

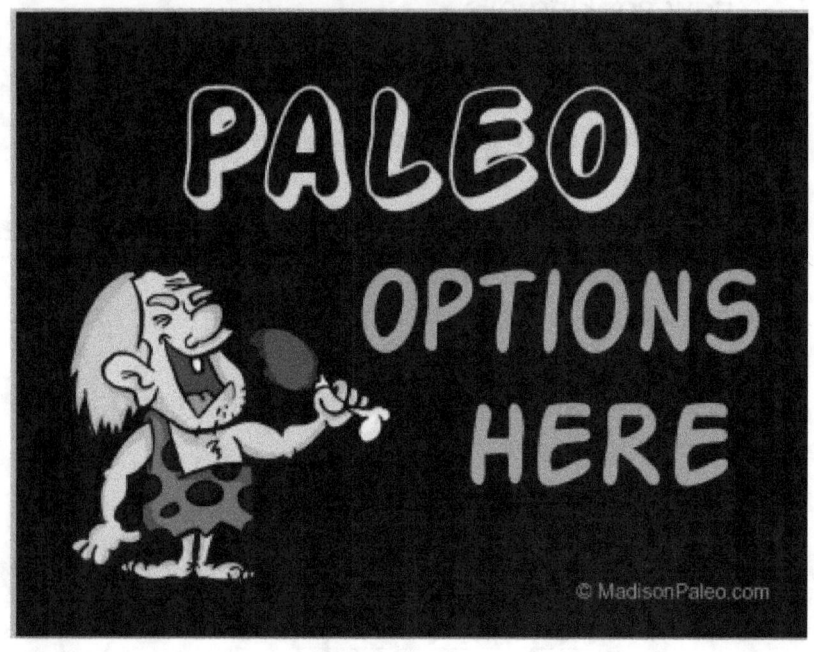

Just email me at servepaleo@gmail.com with a copy of your receipt for this book, and briefly describe what kind of options you offer for paleo diners. (Offer subject to change or cancellation without notice.)

You are also welcome to print this image yourself (if you can do that from the format you're viewing it in) as long as you don't change it, sell it, or remove the copyright notice. You may alter the size to meet your needs. I can make an electronic version of the file available on request.

Guest comments·

"I have worked with a number of eateries, ranging from mom & pop diners to chain restaurants, to integrate "paleo" or gluten free meal options and hygiene practices. An immediate benefit has been a dramatic increase in search engine traffic for these folks as the paleo/gluten free trends are the fastest growing in all of the food industry. The second benefit is gaining a loyal, well networked group of clients who will come back to an establishment that caters to their food needs."

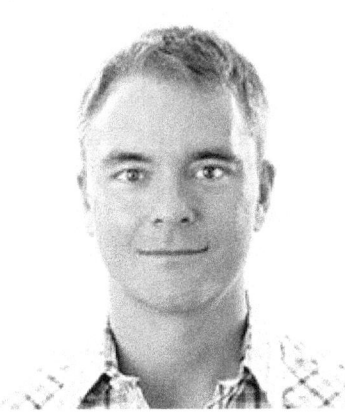

Robb Wolf
Author of <u>The Paleo Solution</u>

www.robbwolf.com

"I've begun creating some grain-free selections to support our customers who are looking for that. We've always had a focus on vegan, vegetarian, and even the very popular gluten-free, but there needed to be more choices offered to our grain-free clientele."

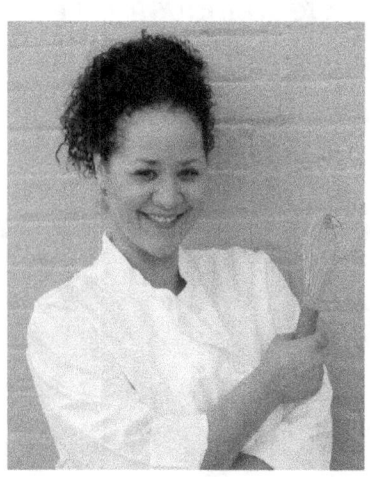

Angelika Matthews
Kitchen Manager and Chef

Willy Street Co-op
Madison, WI
608-251-6776

www.willystreet.coop

"Switching to eating more like our forager-hunter ancestors increases nutrient density, decreases inflammation and is one of the most effective treatments I can offer patients with autoimmune problems, diabetes, obesity, fatigue or early memory loss. Sites like Madison Paleo ("Grain free, dairy free, in the land of fried cheese") can help find dining options for those ready to make the change.

More and more people are learning that medicines may control symptoms for a time, but if they do not address their diet their disease continues to progress. More and more people are turning to food as medicine. The Paleo diet is taking the world by storm. The restaurants that provide more traditional foods, including more organ meats, fermented foods and more non-starchy vegetables as opposed to the grain and white potato based options, will deliver both excellent food and better health. More and more customers will be looking for restaurants that offer Paleo options."

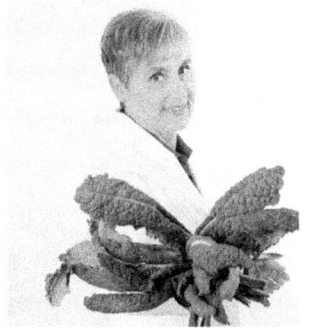

Terry Wahls, M.D.

Author of <u>The Wahls Protocol</u>
www.terrywahls.com

"Since losing 90 pounds, curing lower gastrointestinal bleeding amongst other ailments and feeling better overall, my paleo & primal lifestyle has taken me to where I belong: in the kitchen. I have discovered foods I would have never thought of eating, let alone serving in a restaurant. Let real food be your tour guide and discover a love for cooking that you never knew you had!"

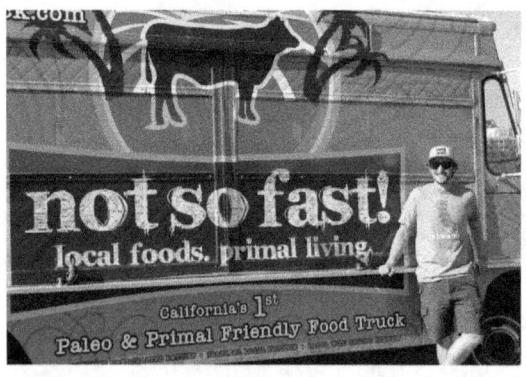

Bob Montgomery

Not So Fast!
Food Truck

San Diego, CA

619-924-9244

www.notsofastfoodtruck.com

"The war on real fats and meat still persists, however cracks in the armor of the low fat, grain based mantra are appearing. More articles and studies are being published routinely now supporting a paleo-style meal plan. The evidence? Bread and soft drink sales are down while real butter sales are up. I would hope that restaurant industry would see that the winds are changing direction and begin to increase the supply of truly 'real foods'."

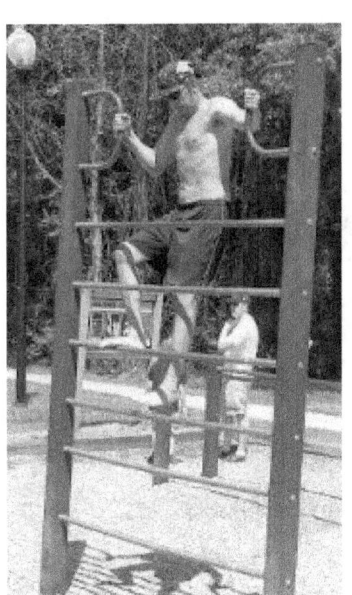

Steve Cooksey

Author of <u>How to Reduce Blood Sugar: The Warrior Way</u>

<u>www.diabetes-warrior.net/</u>

"Eating out while following the Paleo diet can be very tricky, especially if you are craving a sweet dessert at the end of your meal! Let's face it, Paleo or not, many of us are tempted to indulge in something sweet when dining out. Rarely will we find an assortment of desserts free of grains, dairy or refined sugars. However, If restaurants want to cater desserts to the Paleo community, it doesn't have to be complicated.

Simple modifications can be made for so many pre-existing recipes. Desserts that typically include milk or cream could be prepared with coconut milk instead. Refined sugar can easily be replaced with honey. White flour can be replaced with almond flour or coconut flour.

Basic dessert ideas could include:

- seasonal fresh fruit drizzled with honey or topped with whipped coconut milk
- baked apples with cinnamon
- ice creams made with almond milk or coconut milk
- tarts or pies that include a crust made from ground nuts, and sweetened with dates or honey

Offering even one or two safe menu choices for the Paleo community is a great place for restaurants to start. It's not just about catering to a new fad/diet or a specific group of people. It's about providing real food that not only tastes good, but will also contribute to everyone's health and well-being."

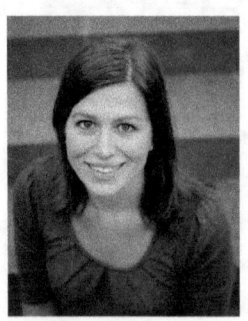

Belle Pleva
Paleo Mama Bakery
Madison, WI
www.paleomamabakery.com

"Food quality is at the root of America's health crisis. Ergo, food quality is also the solution!"

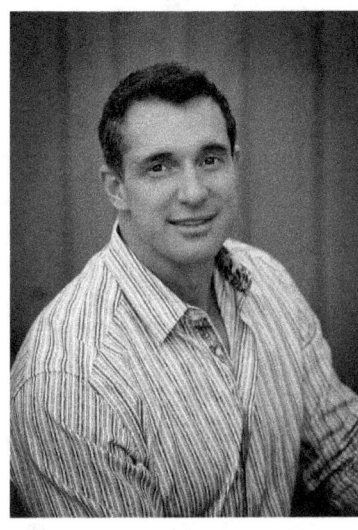

Kirk Parsley, M.D.
@docparsley

www.docparsley.com

"Mission: Heirloom is a one-of-a-kind food company that is revolutionizing the way we eat. We believe that the evolution of healthy food is about more than just organic ingredients. It's about using everything we know about food and health to create nutritious, delicious, and comforting dishes. We meticulously rethink every step in a meal's journey from heirloom seed to the plate, removing layers of toxicity and delivering comforting, replenishing food that satisfies on many levels.

Our culinary process aims to elevate health, elevate food, and elevate joy. Each element on the plate begins with the farmers we know (and love). It continues in a kitchen that's 100% free of gluten, grain, soy, peanuts, and processed food. It culminates with an exotic and deeply satisfying menu centered around nutrient-rich stews and soups, crafted by a team of talented chefs. Along the way we scrupulously avoid kitchen tools and cooking techniques that are potentially harmful.

Like a well tended garden, we are an ever-evolving work-in-progress. We are constantly studying, experimenting, learning, growing, tinkering, and improving. No matter how we grow and expand, our commitment to health and joy will remain unwavering."

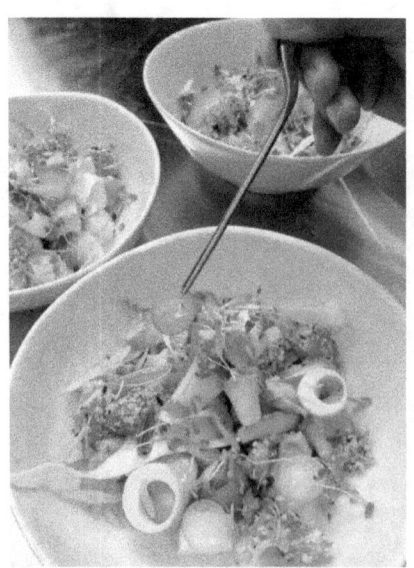

Mission Heirloom
Berkeley, CA

At time of writing, a delivery service and sort of paleo think tank. Plans to open a cafe imminently, and potentially franchise their concept.

http://missionheirloom.com/

Facebook: missionheirloom

"I started my business because there was nothing like it near me. I often say that had a paleo restaurant existed in Indianapolis at the time I would have simply gone and applied for a job instead of starting a company. I wuld like to help other businesses become more paleo friendly by offering consulting. Paleo it forward."

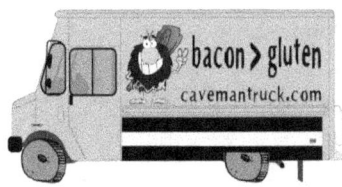

Shelby @ Cavemantruck

http://mkt.com/caveman-truck

317.674.3346

Photo Credits

(Cover) Liver & Onions, paleo style by special request, Capn's Roadhouse, Fort Atkinson, WI - Photo by Joe Disch

Joe teaching "Intro to grain-free diets" at Willy Street Co-op, Madison, WI Photo by Dylan Remis (www.dylanremis.com)

"Uki the caveman" graphic, trademark of Joe Disch and Madison Paleo

Joe with sabertooth skeleton, Vilas Park Zoo, Madison, WI - Photo by Elizabeth Disch

Self-serve hot bar - Photo by Joe Disch

Turkey burgers with spinach salad - Photo by Joe Disch

Making zoodles - Photo by Dylan Remis (www.dylanremis.com)

Cavé - A Paleo Eatery, sign and menu - Photo supplied by subject

Coffee cup - Photo by Joe Disch

Preparation of kale chips - Photo by Joe Disch

Joe's burger with portabella mushroom bun - Photo by Joe Disch

Robb Wolf - Photo supplied by subject

Angelika Matthews of Willy Street Co-op (Madison, WI) - Photo supplied by subject

Terry Wahls, M.D. - Photo by Jonathan D. Sabin

Belle Pleva of Paleo Mama Bakery (Madison WI) - Photo supplied by subject

Bob Montgomery of Not So Fast! Food Truck (San Diego, CA) - Photo supplied by subject

Steve Cooksey of Diabetes-Warrior.net - Photo supplied by subject

Kirk Parsley, M.D. - Photo supplied by subject

Mission Heirloom, Berkeley, CA - Photo supplied by subject

* Guest comments were submitted specifically for this book, and are the opinions of the individual contributors.

www.ingramcontent.com/pod-product-compliance
Lightning Source LLC
Chambersburg PA
CBHW070623290526
45790CB00002B/964

* 9 7 8 1 5 0 2 9 8 3 3 1 2 *